Yoga

Top Yoga Poses
From Beginner to Master

Introduction

I want to thank and congratulate you for downloading the book, "*Yoga: Top Yoga Poses from Beginner to Master*".

This book has actionable information about yoga, as well as some amazing yoga poses that will take you from the beginner level to the pro level.

What comes to mind when you think of yoga? Do you think of it as the impossible stunts that some people pull due to their extreme levels of flexibility like what's shown below?

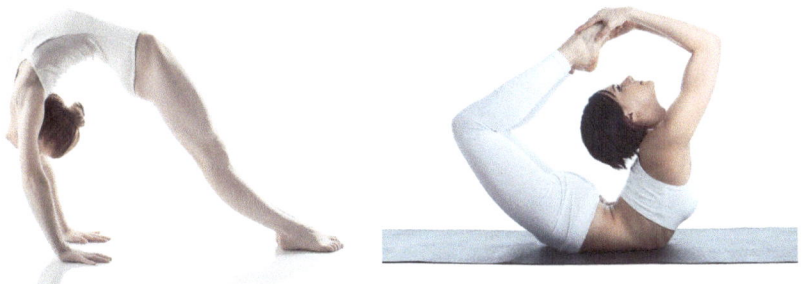

What do you know about it? Do you just think it looks a bit cool to pull these stunts? Do you know that yoga may soon be listed as an Olympic sport? But what exactly is yoga all about? Why is it growing in popularity around the world? Is the growing popularity because of its many benefits? How do you stand to benefit when you do some of these seemingly impossible stunts or asanas)? Do these benefits have any scientific backing? These are just a few of the many questions that you may have about yoga. The good news is that this book will teach you everything you need to know about yoga. It will answer your questions and go a step further to show you how to practice yoga whether you are a complete beginner or an experienced yoga practitioner.

This book will introduce you to some yoga poses, which you can incorporate in your yoga practice. The poses will include poses for beginners, intermediary and master yoga practitioners.

Thanks again for downloading this book, I hope you enjoy it!

Table of Contents

CHAPTER 1

Introduction And Benefits Of
The Concept Of Yoga

What is yoga?

Most people see yoga as a form of physical activity that involves some weird or silly body movements. However, the truth is that yoga transcends the weird movement you notice yoga practitioners pose.

What then is yoga if it is not all about the weight body movements?

Well, yoga is a form of physical and mental exercise. It is a physical activity that involves discipline, mental control, breathing techniques and physical well being. In simpler terms, yoga involves some physical moves, which are combined with mental control and meditation.

A female yoga practitioner is known as a Yogini while a male yoga practitioner is known as a Yogi.

So how did it come into being?

Yoga dates back to over 5000 years ago when it was developed by the Indus-Sarasvati civilization, which was based in Northern India.

The term "yoga" was derived from the word, "Yuj", which literally means to join, to yoke, or to control Sanskrit. When you think of it in terms of the body, mind and soul, yoga portrays the joining of the physical body, mind, and soul or spirit. And when that happens, you are bound to derive a wide array of benefits.

So how is practicing yoga going to benefit you? Let's discuss some of the benefits that you stand to gain through this practice.

Why Yoga?

We have established at this point that yoga transcends a physical movement, but also includes a mental exercise. This means that the benefits of yoga practice will be more than just some physical health benefits. Let us examine some of the benefits of yoga practice.

It Helps in Weight Loss

Although yoga on its own cannot be regarded as an aerobic exercise (exercises that help to increase your heartbeat rate), some athletic types of yoga poses such as the power yoga, the kapal bhati and the sun salutation poses increase your heartbeat, make you sweat and help burn excess fats in the body. So if you are looking for a-not-so strenuous way to burn those excess fats in your body, you should consider making out time to engage in yoga moves daily. The good thing is that you don't need to spend hours on your yoga moves to get results; a 20-minute yoga pose daily can help you achieve your desired result in a short while. Besides weight loss, these athletic yoga poses are also good for people with some serious health issues such as diabetes and high blood pressure. For a diabetic, yoga helps to make the body cells to be more sensitive to insulin in order to regulate the blood sugar level.

It Encourages a Holistic Wellness

Holistic wellness or fitness transcends physical fitness. It involves the emotional and mental well being of your body, mind and soul. The physical postures, meditations, and breathing techniques also known as pranayama give you holistic fitness. Holistic fitness or wellness gives you an inner peace and leads to self realization in the long run.

It Helps to Reduce Stress

Stress can be caused by various factors such as sudden anxiety, or a wide array of physical activities happening around you. One way to cope and reduce stress is by engaging in yoga. This is because the physical poses and breathing techniques associated with yoga serve as a coping mechanism for your body. In addition, yoga helps to relax your body and reduce tensions in the muscles while supplying fresh blood to your brain to keep you vitalized. Finally, it helps to reduce the production of stress-causing hormones, cortisol. Therefore, if you are stressed after your day's activities, you can engage in a quick 20-minute yoga activity to help you relax and have a good night rest.

It helps You Build a Better Relationship

Research has shown that couples that engage in yoga always have a way of building a great relationship. This is because yoga helps to clear your mind, thus helping you to make better decisions on sensitive matters in relationships. Therefore, you can try to get your partner to join your next yoga practice and watch how wonderfully well it will improve your relationship.

It Helps to Build Your Immune System

A low immune system can be caused by many factors such as pollution in the environment and eating the wrong foods. When your immune system is low, your body loses the strength to fight against diseases and this makes you vulnerable to every little disease ranging from flu and cold to other serious illnesses. Yoga helps to boost your immune system by stimulating your lymphatic system to release toxins from your body. In addition, it helps to boost the release of oxygenated blood to your vital body organs to make them work better to fight against antibodies in the body.

It Helps to Boost Your Energy

If you are feeling all tired and weak to face your day, a few minutes of yoga practice may be what you need at that moment. Most advanced yoga poses make you breathe fast and this stretches your chest muscles and allows more air to fill your lungs. This sends the much needed oxygen into your blood, which in turn, revitalizes your body and increases your energy levels. In addition, as I mentioned earlier, yoga helps to reduce the stress-causing hormones and whenever the cortisol level is low, there is always an energy boost and mental alertness in your body.

Obviously, the above list of benefits is not conclusive. Nonetheless, it should have piqued your interest to try yoga to derive some of these and other benefits. The different crazy stunts that you see yoga practitioners pulling are referred to as yoga poses or asanas. To derive the benefits of yoga, you have to implement different asanas. Let us now discuss some yoga moves you can start today to help you enjoy the benefits mentioned above.

CHAPTER 2

Yoga Poses For Beginners

These poses are for beginners. If this is your first time trying out yoga practice, you should start with the easy poses discussed in this chapter. You can move to intermediary poses after you have mastered these ones. One good thing is that these poses for beginners are very easy and can be mastered with great ease.

The Three Legged Downward Dog Pose:

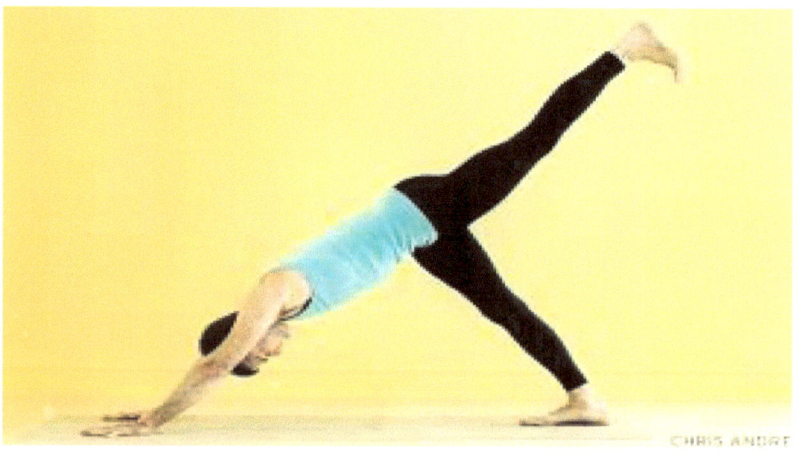

Don't be deceived or discouraged by the long name. This is one of the easiest yoga poses for beginners. This pose is good for strength building especially the training of the arm and shoulder muscles. It also helps to stretch your hips and lower body. This downward facing dog pose is the starting point or basis of many intermediate and advanced poses as you will notice later in this book.

Steps to The 'Three Legged Downward Dog Pose":

- Stand straight with your legs apart.

- Bend until your palms are flat on the floor.

- Slightly stretch out your arms forward and allow your neck to hang lose between your hands.

- Lift your right leg until it gets to the hip point. This creates a 90-degree angle between your two legs.

- Allow your body to relax and concentrate on your breathing.

- When you feel a strain on your arms, bring down your leg and switch to the other leg.

The Upward Facing Dog Yoga Pose:

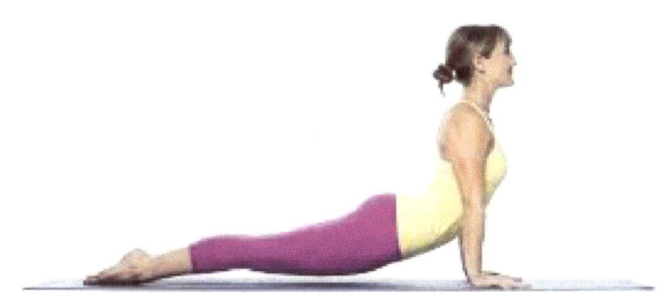

This yoga pose is also known as the urdhva mukha svanasana and it is known as one of the sun salutation yoga poses. You need to do some basic warm-up exercise for your shoulders before you start this yoga pose. While you can do different warm up exercises for this pose, I will suggest the arms circles move.

The Arm Circles Shoulder Warm-up:

- Get into a standing position with your legs wide apart.

- Stretch out your arms on your sides. Get your palms to face the ground.

- Start to rotate your arms in a circular motion 10 times.

- Turn your palms to face upwards and reverse the circular motion.

After the warm up, you can now proceed to the yoga pose.

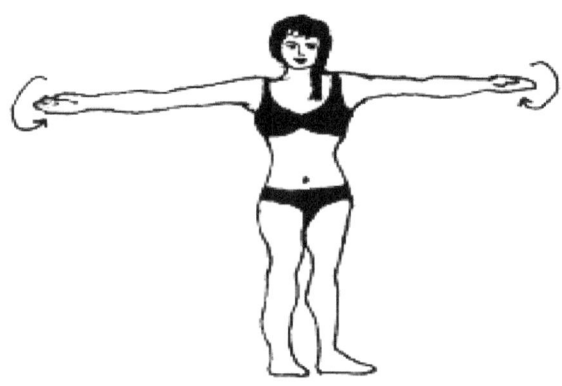

Steps to The "Upward Facing Dog Yoga Pose":

- Lie down on the floor with your head facing the ground.

- Try to lift your body off the floor with your palm firmly placed on the ground.

- You can make it more effective by lifting your hips and thighs totally off the floor i.e. only your feet should touch the floor. This means that you will have to lean heavily on your arm to lift your body off the floor. That was the essence of the shoulder warm-up to help cushion the effect of the weight.

- Try stretching your neck as far back as you can until your face is in an upward direction. This will push out your chest and give your back an arch like shape. Focus on neutral breathing until you feel strain on your arm muscles.

- Relax and repeat.

The Happy Baby Yoga Pose

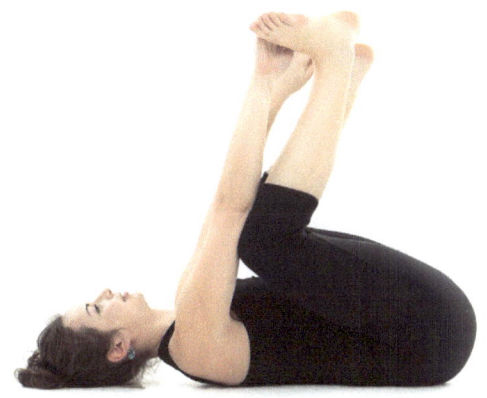

This pose is also called Ananda Balasana yoga pose. It resembles a happy baby in a crib pose. It is meant to unleash the inner baby in you or the innocent part of you because no matter how old you are; you still have this young innocent aspect of your soul. The benefits of this yoga pose include the fact that it helps to strengthen your arms and shoulder muscles. In addition, it helps to relief stress in your body by releasing tension from your lower back. Finally, this pose helps to stretch your outer hips for easier flexibility and your hamstring.

Steps to "The Happy Baby Yoga Pose":

- Lie flat on your back in a comfortable position.

- Bend your knees and place the sole of your feet firmly on the floor.

- Raise your left knee towards your left ankle. Let your right foot remain on the floor.

- Reach across your left shin with your left hand and hold the outside edge of your left foot. If you cannot reach outside your foot, then you can loop a strap over the ball of your left foot and hold it.

- Relax your face and your shoulders, then let your right hand rest on your left hip point and release.

- While still on your back, hold your feet or toes depending on the part of your leg that you can comfortably reach.

- Draw your legs down and roll your butt bones or sit bones and your tailbone toward the floor.

- Stay for a few breaths and repeat.

The Low Lounge Yoga Pose:

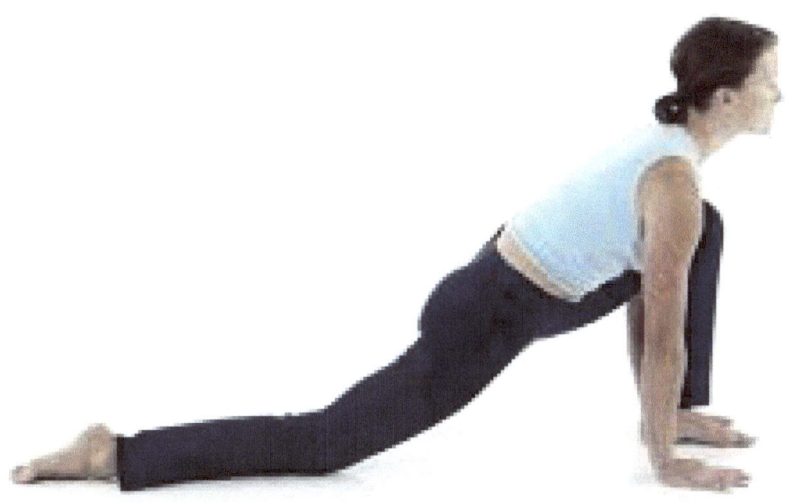

This yoga pose is also called Anjaneyasana. The benefit of this pose is that it stretches your hips, quadriceps, your groins and your hamstring muscles. One good thing about this pose is that it is one of the basic poses for many intermediate or advanced yoga poses.

Steps to "The Low Lounge Yoga Pose":

- Get into downward facing dog pose also known as the Adhomukha Suanasana.

- Take a step forward so that your right foot is placed between your hands.

- Lower your body weight on your left knee and release the top of your left foot on the ground.

- Your right knee should be directly above the right ankle and not moving towards your toes or towards your left or right. This is to avoid any form of knee injury as a result of the weight placed on your knee. One way to know that you got the pose correctly is that you will feel a soothing or comfortable stretch from your groin area straight to your left thigh.

- Place your fingertips on the floor on both sides of your hips. Release your shoulder to go down, away from your ears.

- Focus on your breathing and gently set your body weight to rest on your hips while you draw your tailbone towards the floor.

- Take 10 breaths and release.

- To release or return your normal position, place your toes under, with your hands on the floor.

- Slowly change back to the downward facing dog pose. Take several breaths in the position. Bend your knees and either repeat the pose or release to a standing position.

The Root Bond Yoga Pose

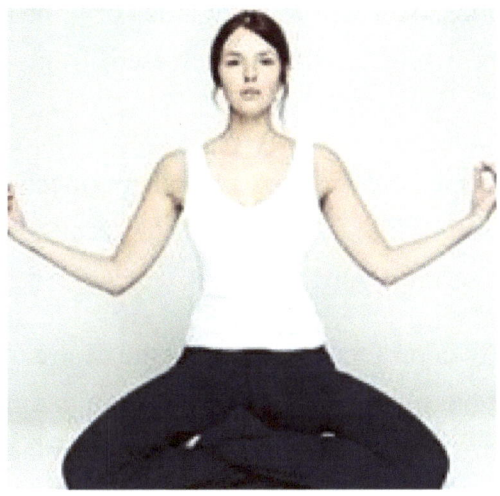

This yoga pose is also referred to as root lock or Muls Bandha. Mula is a translation for root and the idea behind this yoga pose is that it helps you get to your basic torso, which is known as the point of lowest energy centre along your spine column. Some of the benefits of this yoga pose are that it helps you stay calm, boosts your energy levels and aids maximum concentration. Therefore, any time you feel you are feeling fidgety or anxious, you can engage in this yoga pose to calm down your nerves.

Steps to "The Root Bond Yoga Pose":

- Get into a sitting position while keeping your back straight.

- Then cross your legs so that your right foot is tucked or passed under your left knee. The outer side of your foot should touch the floor while the inner side should touch the side of your knee.

- Close your eyes, relax and concentrate on your breathing for a few seconds. You will feel the sides of your rib cage contract and relax while tension is released from your abdominal muscles.

- Then contract the muscles in your perineal region (i.e. your anus region) while you continue to breathe slowly. Continue the exercise until you reach the 20th round.

- Then try to contract the muscles at the centre of your perineum. Contract the muscles tightly without including the urogenital or anal areas. You may stop breathing regularly in the process of trying to get it right.

- Continue with the contraction exercise until you can contract the centre perineal muscles without holding your breathing.

- Stay for 20 seconds and release.

The Garland Yoga Pose

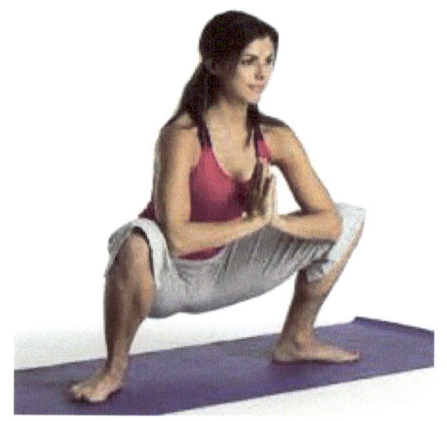

This is another easy yoga pose for beginners. It is also referred to as the Malasana. The benefit of this yoga pose is that it helps to tone up your abdominal region i.e. your abs. It also helps to stretch your back, ankles and groin.

Steps to "The Garland Yoga Pose":

- Get into a squat position and keep your feet close together.

- Your heels should remain on the floor or you can place them on a folded yoga mat for support.

- Separate the thighs in a position so that it becomes wider than the torso. Then lean the torso forward and proceed to fit it between your thighs.

- Place your elbow on your inner knees with your palms together in an Anjali Mudra or salutation seal position. That is placing your palms together as though you are praying or making a supplication.

- Finally, resist your knees into your elbow.

- You can advance it a bit by bringing your inner thighs to press against the sides of your torso. Then bring your arm forward and swing to the sides.

- Place your fingertips on the floor and grasp the back heel. Stay put for 1 minute and straight out your knees.

- Exhale and slowly stand.

There are many other yoga poses for beginners but these ones are the very easy poses you can master in no time. After you master the beginner's poses, you may want to take up something more challenging. In that case, you can start with the intermediary yoga poses. The next chapter will detail some more advanced or challenging yoga poses.

CHAPTER 3

The Intermediate Yoga Poses

In this chapter, I will discuss four common yoga poses for intermediary yoga practitioners.

The Standing Split Yoga Pose:

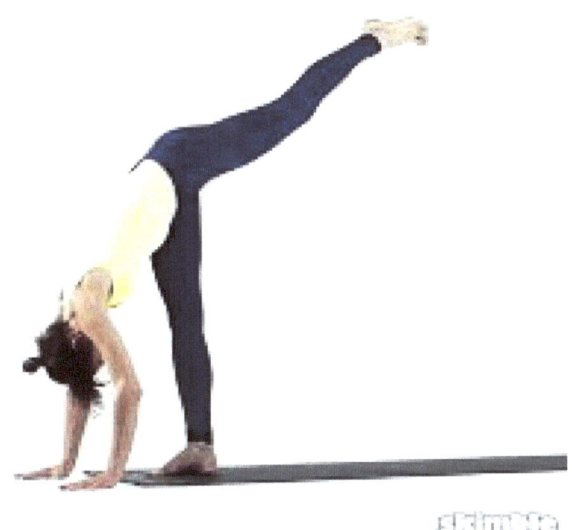

This yoga pose is also called the Urdhva Prasarita Eka Padasana, which can be literally translated to mean 'one foot extended upward'. Some of the benefits of this yoga pose are that it helps to stimulate your liver and kidney. It strengthens your knees, ankles, back of your legs and groin region.

Steps to "The Standing Split Yoga Pose":

- Get into a Warrior II yoga pose as shown in the image below.

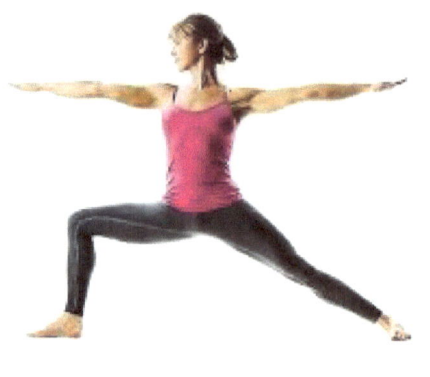

JASPER JOHAL

- Start a cartwheel position with your right arm above your head to create an opening on your right ribs.

- Twist your torso to the left. Lean a bit forward and place your palms on the floor.

- Lean the front of your torso to your left thigh. Take two steps ahead with your hands and shift your body to your left foot.

- Slowly straighten your left leg as you lift your right leg to become parallel to the floor. This process should be done simultaneously.

- Try to raise your raised leg a little bit higher. Stay for 1 minute and lower your raised leg. Exhale and repeat the exercise or get to a standing position.

The One Legged Pigeon Pose:

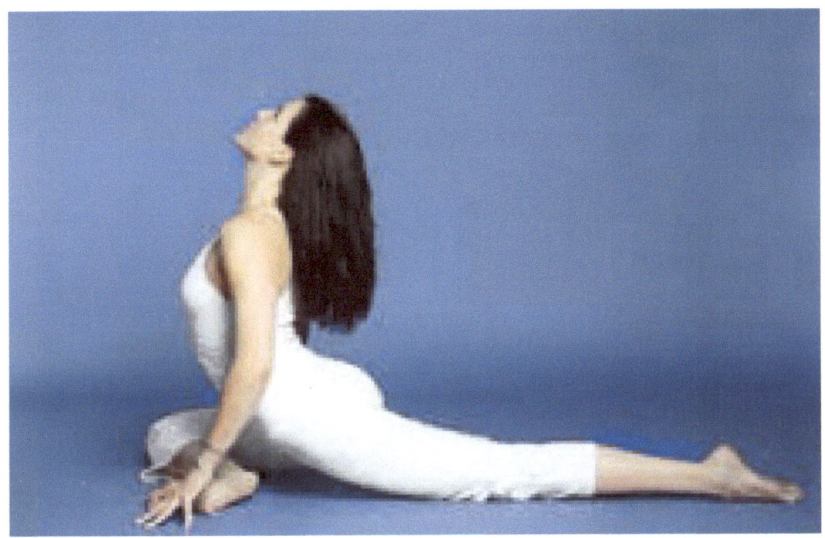

This pose is also known as the pigeon pose or the Eka Pada Rajaka Potasana. The benefit of engaging in this yoga pose is that it helps to open up your hip joints, increases your flexibility and serves as a quick relief for anxiety or stress. It is worth mentioning at this point that the pigeon yoga pose is not recommended for you if you are pregnant. It is also not suitable for persons with ankle or knee injuries. This yoga pose involves putting some pressure on your knees and ankles so any injury or pain on those areas will only get worse. That is why it is recommended that people with knee and ankle injuries should avoid this particular pose until their injury is perfectly healed.

Steps to "The One Legged Pigeon Pose":

-     Get into the downward facing dog yoga pose.

- Bring your left knee between your hands and place your left ankle near your right wrist.

- Extend your right leg behind you in such a way that your kneecap and your foot rest well on the floor.

- Place your palms on the floor and lift your torso away from your thigh.

- Bring down your front leg and place your body weight balanced on your right and left hips. Slide down softly and remain in the position for about 10 seconds.

- Get back to the downward facing dog pose and repeat the pose.

The Extended Hand-to-Big-Toe Yoga Pose:

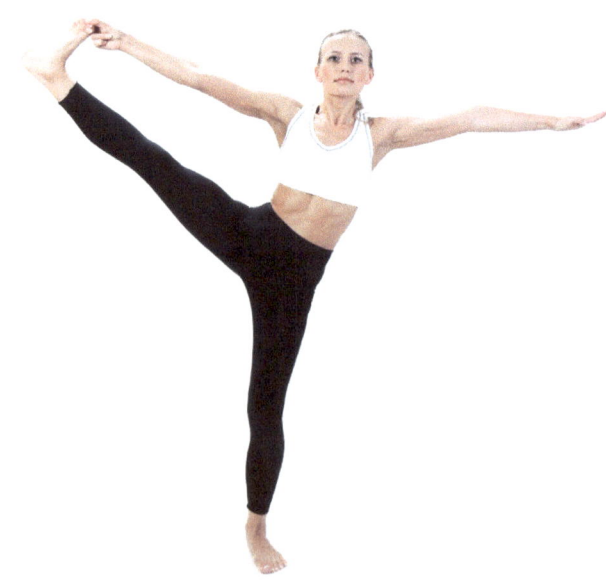

This pose is also known as the Utthita Hatsa Padangustasuna. The benefit of this pose is that it helps you develop deep concentration and stay calm. It also stretches your legs and hamstring muscles. This yoga pose is also not recommended for a pregnant woman or for people with knee or ankle injuries because of the reasons I stated earlier.

Steps to "The Utthita Hasta Padangustasuna":

- Stand with your legs closed and your hands on your sides (this is called the mountain pose).

- Take several deep breaths and shift your body weight to your left leg.

- Lift your right leg off the ground and stretch it out in front of you in such a way that it becomes parallel to the ground.

- Place your hand on your hips for support and slowly move your leg until it is stretched out by your side.

- Stretch your right hand to touch your foot without bending sideways.

- Continue with the position for a minute, go back to the mountain pose and repeat on the other leg.

The Big Toe Yoga Pose

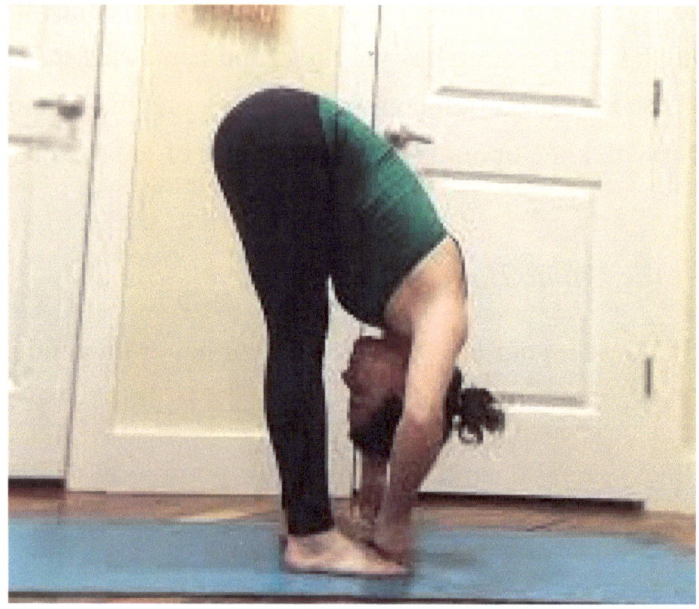

This is another form of doing the pose, which I just explained earlier. It is called the Padangusthasana.

Steps to "The Big Toe Yoga Pose"

- Stand with your legs slightly apart, about 10 inches apart.

- Keep your legs straight and bend your hips until your palm is placed on the floor. Lean towards the floor to allow your elbows bend outward.

- Grab your big toe on each of your hands and allow your neck to hang lose

- Concentrate on your breathing, for 20 seconds, then exhale and release.

CHAPTER 4

The Advanced Or Masters Yoga Pose

These are more advanced poses and require some level of flexibility on your part to master it well.

The Firefly Yoga Pose:

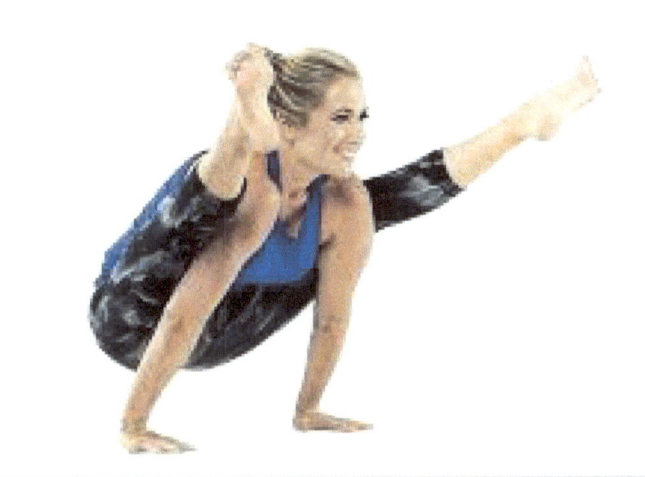

This pose is also known as the Tittibhasana, which is a Hindu name for insect. This yoga exercise helps to open up your chest and gives you strength and flexibility.

Steps to "The Firefly Yoga Pose":

- Get into The Uttanasana pose as shown in the image below

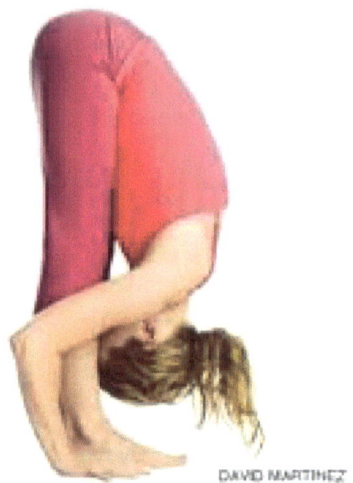

- Place your shoulder behind your legs. Bring your knees together, then squeeze and bend your knees.

- Place your hand on the floor behind your heels. Lean your body weight on your hands and squeeze your knees towards each other.

- Push your shoulder back to your knee to give your shoulder some form of stability.

- Your hands should remain on the floor while you tighten your kneecaps and lift yourself off the floor. Hold for 10 seconds and release.

An Easier Method is:

- Sit on the floor with your butt.

- Place your legs on top of your arms.

- Then lean forward and lift your butt and legs off the floor.

The Peacock Yoga Pose:

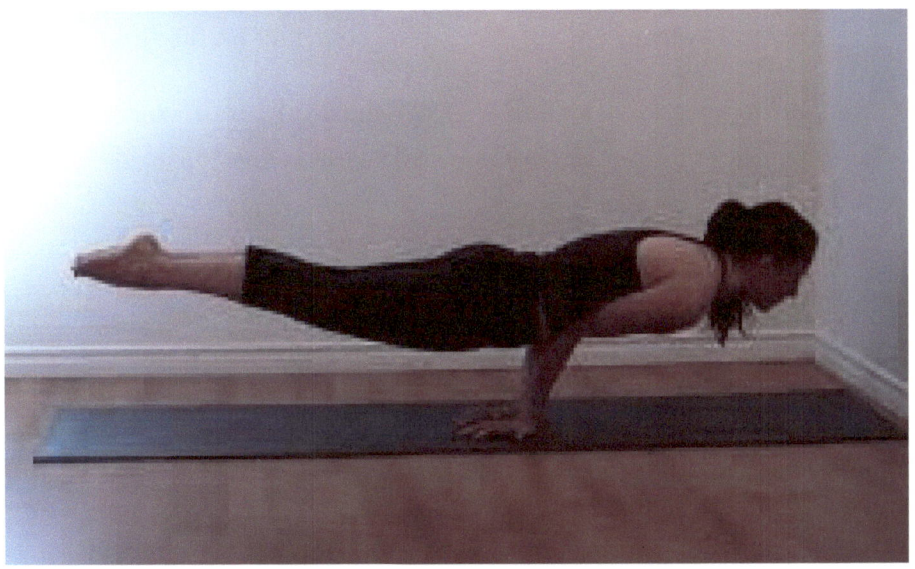

This is also referred to as the Mayurasana.

Steps to "The Peacock Yoga Pose":

- Kneel on the floor with your knees wide part.

- Sit on your heels and lean forward a bit.

- Place your palms on the floor and turn your fingers back to face your torso.

- Bend your elbows outside and touch your outer forearm with your small finger.

- Bend your elbows to the outside of your arms and lean your torso to your back.

- Firm your abdomen against your elbow. Stretch your legs behind your torso with the top of your feet on the floor.

- Firm up and lift your legs off the floor until your legs are parallel to the floor. Hold for 10 seconds and release.

The Tortoise Yoga Pose

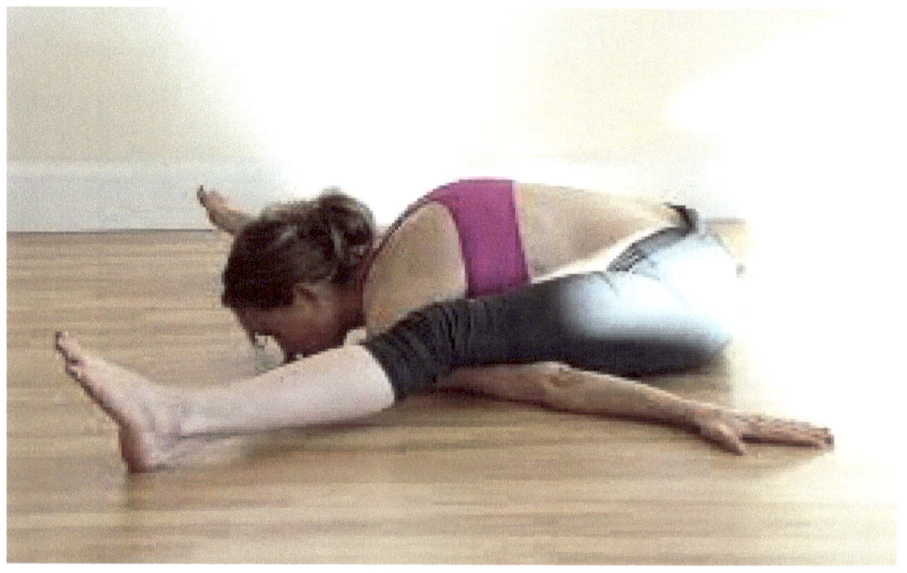

It is also known as the Kurmasana. It helps to calm your mind, increase flexibility, strengthens your back and tones your abs.

YOGA

Steps to "The Tortoise Yoga Pose":

- Get into the downward facing dog pose

- Spread your legs as apart as you can. Bend your knees a little and place your arms under your knees.

- Continue to stretch out the arms until they reach behind your back.

- Stretch out your legs and pull your shoulders to the floor. Allow your forehead or jaw to touch the floor.

- Stay for 10 seconds and get back to the downward facing dog position.

Conclusion

Again, many thanks for downloading this book!

I hope this book was able to help you understand how to implement different yoga poses to derive different benefits.

The next step is to implement what you've learnt.

Finally, if you enjoyed this book, would you be kind enough to leave a review for this book on Amazon?

Go to the link below to leave a review for this book on Amazon!

http://www.amazon.com/Yoga-Beginner-Relaxation-Mindfulness-Self-Esteem-ebook/dp/B01DE6M68K

Thank you and good luck!

www.ingramcontent.com/pod-product-compliance
Lightning Source LLC
Chambersburg PA
CBHW050909290526
45792CB00002B/757